Clean Eating:

The Essential Guide to Eating Clean including Recipes and Meal Plan. NOW, with Tips and Hints for KIDS!

by Josh West

Table of Contents

Introduction:

I want to thank you for purchasing this book: "Clean Eating".

This book contains proven steps and strategies on how to become a truly healthy person by eating clean. When you eat clean you feel more focused and energetic. With patience and the help of this book it will become second nature for you to fill your shopping basket with wholesome foods and leave the processed foods on the shelf.

Many of our favorite foods are packed with unnecessary chemical preservatives and fillers, to increase "shelf life." Additionally, you may live in a neighborhood where you will find foods on your grocery shelf that have been grown using genetically modified organisms (GMOs), or other technologies to increase shelf life. Much of what we consume today can hardly be described as food! One key way to identify what is a "clean food" and what is not, is to remember; if it's raw or unprocessed, it will most likely be clean.

Before we begin, you might want to take stock of what you have in your kitchen pantry. Sit down and make a list of the items that you use on a regular basis to feed your family. Then, with the help of this book, you will find healthy, clean alternatives, and be on your way to becoming the amazing healthy person you are by eating clean!

Chapter 1: What is Clean Eating?

You may have heard this phrase tossed around the local health food aisle, but what is clean eating? How do you eat clean? The first thing you need to keep in mind, as you read this book, is that you cannot attain your weight loss or health goals without using clean eating as the foundation. You can exercise as much as you physically can; however, if you go through your favorite drive through for greasy foods afterwards, or continue to buy highly processed foods when you shop, you aren't going to lose anything and your body is still going to be in the same unhealthy condition. The types of food you eat directly affects your health and weight in significant ways. If you eat healthy; focusing on whole, raw and other fresh foods, your skin and body will glow with amazing health, giving you boundless energy and vitality.

The Basic Principals of Eating Clean

There are a few basic principles to "eating clean." In this section, we examine a few of these principles, concentrating on what makes each unique; but, always with a focus on what makes each principal a healthy alternative.

The First Principal

Read labels!

The first principal to eating clean is to avoid all chemicals, GMO's, additives, preservatives, and any unnatural ingredients. These are normally referred to as "fake foods." They lack the nutritional value you need to live a healthy life, and they seem to rule the grocery stores nowadays.

The next time you go to your local market, take a moment to simply look at the packaging, read and understand how pervasive highly processed foods have become. Most of the shelves are stocked with these unhealthy choices. Take a moment to read the labels. You will be stunned by what we consume as food. Other than the fresh produce, or items that are clearly marked as "organic" pretty much all the items in your local market are highly processed and filled with the chemicals and additives that make us sick. Most of us would like to avoid these types of foods and improve our health. We may not necessarily be looking to lose any weight, but we all want to improve our health and increase our vitality by avoiding the fake factory processed foods.

Take a long close look at the ingredient list of any processed food you use on a regular basis. You will see many different substances that are added to the foods you eat simply to increase shelf-life or make them look more appetizing. Here is a partial list of processed foods and their alternative "clean" choices that will help you better pinpoint what should be on your shopping list.

DAIRY

Milk is the most basic of processed foods and widely used by families around the word as a daily commodity in their diet. Milk was originally processed to increase shelf-life. And, as we moved from a rural, to an urban/industrial society milk producers have lowered the health benefits of milk as they have increased yield and shelf-life. Whole milk has been slowly transformed into something that is good for you, into something filled with allergens and carcinogens.

In modern milk production, cows are fed a combination of high protein and soy based feeds instead of grass and hay. These feeds along with modern breeding techniques, give the animals abnormally large pituitary glands and increases milk production. In return, the animals need large amounts of antibiotics to keep them healthy. These antibiotics end up in the milk we drink. Additionally, synthetic Vitamin D is added to replace the natural Vitamin D found in milk fat, which is removed in the homogenization process. In addition, BGH (Bovine Growth Hormone) is often added to the animals' and has been shown to cause cancer.

These are only a few of the "dirty" problems found with modern milk production. But, alternatives to milk; like Almond, Soy, Cashew and Coconut milk are not always a clean substitute either.

Carrageenan is a produce made from red seaweed, is natural and found in many of these milk substitute products, including products marked "organic." Most Carrageenan found in these products degrade in the body, in the gastrointestinal tract and liver, where it can cause inflammation and intestinal abnormalities. A great deal has been written about soy and its use in milk. Additionally, many of these products have cane sugar added for taste.

So, what can we do to buy and use healthy milk products?

Think raw. It is not always easy to find, but "raw" milk is the best alternative. Goat milk and cheese is also a good choice in that goat farming doesn't have many of the issues found in industrial cow milk production?

Eating yogurt, especially natural yogurt cultures like those found in Organic Greek yogurts are a great solution for your daily dairy needs.

Remember, eating clean is eating smart. Read the labels on the food you buy, and make informed choices for you and your family.

GRAINS; BREAD, PASTA AND PROCESSED GRAINS

The essential thing we want to remember when choosing grains to eat is whole grains versus processed grains. The growing and consuming of grains has been a part of the essential dietary product of human civilization since the invention of agriculture.

While the eating of grains is elementary to our diets, the advent of processed grains is basically a result of trying to answer the question of how do we use technology and the industrialization of the modern food chain to feed large populations. Thus, the breads and pastas that have become popular in the market place are made with processed, "enriched" wheat flour.

Enriched white flour and the products made from it are enriched by adding vitamins and nutrients back into the flour that have been stripped from the grain because of modern processing. Now, instead of eating a whole grain that is digested slowly, giving you access to the natural complex sugars which are slowly digested in the body and high fibers which are essential for good digestive health, we are eating simple sugars that burn quickly or stored as fat, leaving us hungry and contributing to a wide variety of illnesses and problems; like, obesity, arthritis, heart disease, allergies, gluten intolerance and more.

These days there is a wide variety of grains available for you to consume. Brown breads and pastas are plentiful in the markets, but even those need to be used cautiously. Read the labels. Some whole wheat (Brown) breads and pastas have additives.

As the awareness for clean eating has improved, and more information has been released about the health problems that come with eating enriched gains, some of the lesser known "legacy" grains have gained notoriety in the market place. Barley, Oat, Millet, Quinoa, and Rye, are just some of these legacy whole grains that are better for you than enriched wheat or even whole wheat (brown) flour and contribute to good health and increased energy. Some of them are harder to use, but the benefits out way any inconvenience you may experience.

Likewise, raw grains and nuts have much more nutrients and vitamins available for you in your breakfast or snacking.

Think: the crunchier, the better.

FRUITS AND VEGETABLES

Clean eating is not about diets; it is about a life-style change. Moving from foods that are processed and adulterated with fillers, preservatives and synthetic nutrients to fresh and raw foods is a commitment to change in your life style. This is about eating in the way our bodies were meant to consume food for the body's optimum benefit.

What is more natural to eat than fresh foods and vegetables? Nothing. Basic rule of thumb in eating clean; load up on fresh fruits and vegetables. Our bodies are made for it.

The health benefits from eating fresh fruits and vegetables is well known. Eating a diet rich in fruit and vegetables can help reduce the risk of heart disease, stroke, cancer and type-2 diabetes, among many other ailments and diseases. Fruits have no cholesterol. Fruits and vegetables are high in potassium which can lower blood pressure, and are a nature source of dietary fiber which helps digestion and promotes a healthy gut.

Certain fruits, such as grapes (the grape seed and skin) and blue berries are high in a substance known as bioflavonoid. Bioflavonoids are a family of nutrient chemical compounds that help in the absorption of Vitamin C, support blood circulation and are a group of powerful anti-oxidants that help in aging.

You want to try vegetables that are rich in color; purple, yellow, and green; Red Cabbage, Kale, Squash and Egg Plant for example. These colorful vegetables have higher amounts of the essential vitamins and minerals you need. Steam your vegetables or eat them raw to gain the greatest benefit from the produce you consume. When you over cook your vegetables, you remove the nutrients.

Wash ALL fruits and vegetables before eating. Some have been subjected to chemical insecticides. One way to avoid chemical insecticides is to only buy Organic. However, even organically grown fruits and vegetables can be exposed to the salmonella bacteria during the growing process and cause food poisoning when eaten. Wash your fruits and vegetables before eating.

While it is important to eat fruits and vegetables daily, be careful in how much fruit you consume. Remember, fruits are broken down into sugars. Complex carbohydrates such as fructose (the sugars found in fruit) can also cause problems. Too much sugar, even natural ones, can be a problem.

Balance and moderation. Everything is a process of balance, moderation and finding the right amount/combination of raw/clean foods that are best for you.

EATING CLEAN PROTEIN

When we think about eating protein, we normally think; beef, chicken and fish. And, while these are good sources of protein in an average diet, there are many problems around eating meat as your main source of protein that you need to consider if you are trying to maintain "clean eating" habits.

The problems with most protein derived from meats are, again, a result of the modern industrial processes used to raise the animals. From the anti-biotics and hormones added to the feed of most beef, hog and chickens to the heavy metals such as mercury found in fish.

When choosing meat protein for your meals you want to look for packaging that is clearly labeled with language such as; "Hormone Free", "No Anti-Biotics Used", "Free Range" or "Organic". Looking for meats that have phrases such as these on their packaging will help you avoid meats containing antibiotics, hormone or the heavy metals. But, even a steady diet of meat, can still cause problems. Eating meat high in animal fat can contribute to cholesterol; which leads to heart disease. Depending on how you cook your meats, there are potential issues with Cancer.

There are other sources of Protein

Beans and Legumes are a great source of dietary protein and are high in fiber, calcium, and iron. They should be included as part of your "rotation" of foods you regularly buy and consume.

Tofu, soy beans, lentils, split peas, peanuts and mongo beans are only a few of the many beans and legumes that are readily available at your neighborhood grocery, are easy to prepare and can provide you with your daily intake of dietary protein.

If you eat prepared meats, make sure they are cooked all the way through. Also, prepare meals using simply cooked meats. For example, chicken with only a dash of seasoning. Or, beef with a few sprinkles of pepper. We often prepare meat dishes that are smothered with rich sauces that only add to our overall fat intake. Put that nice chicken breast on the grill with a brushing of olive oil and some cayenne.

Chapter 2: Tips and Tricks for Clean Eating

If the concept of "clean eating" sounds complicated and expensive, it is only as problematic as you make it. At its heart, "clean eating" is about making conscious, healthy choices in the way you eat. At its core, this is a strategy about eating unaltered, unprocessed and raw foods. It's about treating yourself as good as you can and realizing that you can live a healthier life by eating in a simple and clean way. The adage; "you are what you eat" could not be more true.

In this chapter, we want to share a few tips and tricks for clean eating so you can make better choices when you shop at popular grocery stores.

Clean Eating and Lowering Your Cost

Clean eating may seem like an expensive proposition for you and your family. It doesn't have to be that way. Families often avoid clean eating due to the misconception that clean eating costs too much money. However, there is a way to provide good clean food options for a larger sized family or one that simply needs to save money on groceries.

Most processed foods cost more than raw or foods with simple ingredients.

Bulk Shop

Begin your quest for clean foods in the bulk item section of your local health food or popular grocery store. Try shopping in bulk, stock up on the raw clean foods you like. Items like; beans, whole grains, barley, quinoa, millet, and whole grain flours are usually available in bulk.

One item that you want to watch for in purchasing in bulk is salt. Choose natural sea salts. Another thing to remember about bulk items you purchase; they are usually fresh. But be careful when you buy in bulk that you don't purchase more than you will use. Bulk items can go stale or turn rancid. Bulk items, especially products that are organic, will not have any additives to ensure freshness. Make sure you are buying fresh, or the "sell by" date is clearly marked on the bin. Get to know your grocer. Ask questions.

The Trials and Tribulations of Eating Organic, Vegan, Gluten-free, etc.

The reason why eating organic has become so popular is in the list of ingredients you find on must food packaging. Eating "Organic" is eating cleaner, but it does not necessarily mean "eating clean." The entire concept of organic farming is to encourage soil and water conservation. Organic farmers use natural fertilizers sophisticated crop rotation techniques and mulch to control weeds. And, food products with the certification of "Organic" meet these standards. However, it doesn't' mean they are always free of fillers and other ingredients to assure freshness and improve shelf-life.

Produce and Vegetables with the certification of "100% Organic" are the cleanest produce available, but packaged foods with added ingredients need to be given a second look at the label to make sure they don't contain additives that can cause allergic reactions or other potential health related problems like Gluten or Milk intolerance. Be suspicious of packaging that claims to be "Natural" or "All Natural" or "Hormone Free." Again, read the labels. Make sure the ingredients match up with the claims. If you have questions, ask the employees at the story where you shop. Educate yourself on all those odd sounding words found on labels.

The good news, more and more "organic" products can found on the shelves of your neighborhood grocery store. You no longer need to shop only at higher priced "organic" and "natural foods" specialty markets. But, it does mean you need to be a more discerning shopper. We can't say it enough, read labels.

The "Skinny" on Saturated Fats

There has been a great deal written and many studies conducted on the issue of fat in the modern diet. The rule of thumb for a long time now is that unsaturated fats in moderation are good for you and saturated fats are not. New studies and science is painting a subtler picture. The goal is still the same, eat foods that include good fats like nuts and seeds and their oils which are low in bad cholesterol (LDL) and promote healthy cholesterol (HDL).

Eating fish and consuming foods high in Omega-3s are fatty

foods which are good for you. However, again, make sure the fish you eat are from sources which are clean and absent of feed additives and any heavy metals that might be found in the fish.

Eating foods cooked with Olive oil, or other oils high in Omega-3s such as Grapeseed, Almond or Peanut oil are also a great way to get the fat in your diet that you need. But, even with these healthy oils watch out of contamination. The oils can go bad, become rancid. Butter from grass fed animals can be rich in healthy fats, but beware of processed butters and margarines, they are high in those unhealthy LDL fats.

Absolutely avoid Canola, Corn and Soybean oils. Not only are they exceedingly high in LDLs, they are almost always sourced from crops that are use GMOs.

Like everything else in your pursuit to eat clean, read the labels.

Cook from "Scratch"

Everyone has a busy life these days. To make our lives easier, the market shelves are filled with pre-packaged meals that you simply need to open and heat up in the microwave or dump into a skillet to heat up and serve. In almost every case, those prepackage meals are filled with the same added ingredients you are trying to avoid.

There are ways you can use some prepackaged food items as a clean base to whip up a delicious and clean meal for your family. One of the easiest solutions for a clean meal on a busy day are prepackaged salads. They have become very popular and are found in many grocery store produce sections. They contain very few fillers and ingredients to increase shelf-life (read the labels of any prepackaged dressings) and should include a "sell by" date on the packaging which will help you determine freshness.

Another prepackaged item that can help are frozen vegetables. Toss the frozen vegetables in a skillet with a little olive oil, garlic, sea salt and a little pepper, add a bit of diced chicken and you've quickly created a clean meal. By simply adding a little precooked protein to the packaged salad or frozen vegetables, you have yourself a pretty quick and relatively clean meal for you or your family.

Another strategy you might try is pre-cooking several "clean meals" ahead of time and storing them in the freezer. Try this the next time you bring home a nice tray of chicken breasts, pork cutlets or lean ground beef. Cook them up all at once with a little seasoning. Cut up some to add into your salads or other meals to use as needed. Leave a few whole cooked chicken breasts or lean hamburger patties in a storage container in your refrigerator for a quick pick me up. In our house, we call these burger or chicken "cookies." You're a little hungry with no time? Grab a burger cookie from the refrigerator and go. Either with a quick warm up from the microwave or eaten cold, you've given yourself a boost of energy from clean protein and are on your way.

Tips on How to Start Clean Eating

When you think of getting started on clean eating, think simple. Like any new idea you take on, change can be daunting. It's easier to continue eating and doing what we have always done. To change is a challenge. The best way to take this new idea of Clean Eating is to take it "one bite at a time."

Whenever we decide to change our lives, we should be kind to ourselves. Commit to the change and give yourself space to fail. Old habits die hard and we can find ourselves in the frustrating position of not meeting our new standards and then dropping our attempt to improve our lives because we believe we can't do it. You can do it. If you believe it, it will happen.

To begin your adventure in clean eating, start by choosing just one meal a day to eat in this new clean way. Give yourself an easy win and build upon that success. As an example, try a breakfast of fruit and organic Greek yogurt with a dash of honey and cinnamon. Change that up by adding a bit of Granola or another unrefined grain or whole nuts. Spend the first week of your quest for clean eating trying a variety of combinations of clean produce, dairy and grain.

Keep the ingredients simple. Use spices and herbs for your flavoring. This is the time to try out a vegetable that you have never heard of before. Stick to the very basics and keep the meals basic. Think about broccoli, chicken breasts, and some brown rice. Once you have gotten the hang of it, you can then branch out.

Pick a few easy recipes from this book that you would like to try out for the week. Trying one or even two recipes every week will enable you to begin to get the hang of the new way of cooking without getting completely overwhelmed.

Plan for leftovers. This will make your lunchtime much easier. You can even do this for your dinner.

Make a list of some snacks that you like that are clean; i.e. nuts, dried fruits, popcorn, etc.

Every week, when you go grocery shopping, switch out one of the ingredients that you would normally purchase for something new. For example, once the white pasta has run out, replace the pasta with a yellow spaghetti squash and try your regular Bolognese sauce with this new substitute.

If you do not already have a small cooler, you will need to get one so that you can carry your lunches, snacks, and dinner with.

Create an emergency kit for clean eating in your car and at work. This kit should include clean foods that you can eat if you forgot your food or something else has happened. Some good items are protein bars (beware of protein bars with Corn Syrup in them), nuts, dry oats, and dried fruits with no sugar added. These are great clean food items you can keep in your car for those "Hungry" moments.

You will need to expect and plan for the mistakes. Making some mistakes is more a type of frame of mind than anything else. If you know that you will make mistakes, get off track, you can plan for them. They will not completely derail your efforts. nIf you find that you have purchased or even eaten something that is not clean, just ensure that you do better the next meal. This frame of mind will ensure that clean eating will become a habit.

Chapter 3: Hints for Kids

Kids can, and should eat clean as well. If you are a busy parent, it's easy to include your children in what you are preparing for the family. But, what about those food products that are targeted to children? Again, read labels and look for added sugar. Obesity in children is a serious problem today. Be on the lookout the phrase; "High Fructose Corn Syrup." This is a product derived from corn and is a horrible product for your children to consume. You find it in candies and all manner of "sweet" products. It is usually added to all those box juices and fruit roll-ups you see in the stores for children. Make sure you are buying products for your children that contain "Whole Juice". Beware of packaging that claims to contain "Natural Sweeteners." High Fructose Corn Syrup is a natural sweetener. It is also the worst ingredient you can feed to your children. Be very careful of products that claim to have no "High Fructose Corn Syrup." Read the label. Ingredients like HFCS90 or "Regular" HFCS are still corn syrup and bad for your children.

Kids can be fickle when it comes to what they eat. Luckily, you can plan for their pickiness. In this chapter, you are going to learn how to ensure that you kids are eating clean. Getting your family to eat a clean and healthy way can be extremely tough. Despite your insistence on this diet, kids will still want those Frosted Pop Tarts and those greasy burgers. A parent's persistence and the kid's growing awareness of different food will potentially provide fuel to their clean eating. However, you will learn some ways to get your little ones eating clean.

- Stock the kitchen with some healthy, convenient foods. These foods include:
  - ✓ Apples
  - ✓ Strawberries
  - ✓ Grapes
  - ✓ Pineapple
  - ✓ Celery
  - ✓ Cauliflower
  - ✓ Broccoli
  - ✓ Pecans
  - ✓ Walnuts
  - ✓ Almonds
  - ✓ Rice Cakes
  - ✓ Dried Fruit
  - ✓ Unsweetened Applesauce

- Trash the white and buy the brown flour rice, bread, etc. Kids love bread, as long as it is soft. If your kids prefer white rice and you find it difficult to do the switch, then you can begin by mixing the brown into the white rice. Little by little take out the white.

- Add extra vegetables in your recipes. A recipe for some tasty smashed potatoes includes mashed cooked cauliflower mixed with mashed potatoes. Another recipe adds in cooked and mashed carrots into the tomato sauce for a baked pasta dish. Your family may be able to tell something is a bit different, but they will not mind it.

- Bake some healthy snacks. When kids reach the teen years, they will need some extra protein. It is a good idea to make some protein bars and then use baggies to store them. You can make Applesauce Protein Bars, which is a hit with most kids. Here is a quick overview of the recipe:

  - ✓ You will need: 1 cup whey protein powder, ½ cup of spelt flour, 2 cups of rolled oats, ½ cup of oat bran, ½ cup of flax seed, 1 tsp. Of sea salt, 1 tsp. Of cinnamon, ½ tsp. Of allspice, ¼ tsp. Of nutmeg, ¼ tsp. Of pepper, ¼ cup of agave nectar, 1 ½ cup of unsweetened applesauce, ¼ cup of safflower oil, and 1 Tbsp of vanilla.
  - ✓ In order to make the bars you will need to mix all of the dry ingredients together, and then all of the wet ingredients together. Mix in the wet ingredients to the dry ones, and then bake is inn a 9 x 13 pan for 20 to 25 minutes on 325 degrees Fahrenheit.

- Embrace the snack time in order to encourage healthy foods. Make the snacks fun, along with healthy.

- Eat nut butters that are natural rather than commercial peanut butters. Commercial peanut butter will raise your cholesterol. If you purchase natural peanut butter your cholesterol will go down.

- Do not purchase the sugared cereal. If the option is not there, then they will not eat it. Bran cereals are delicious, especially when you add natural honey to it as a sweetener.

- Understand that you kids will not love every single fruit or vegetable that you try to feed them. As long as you work with them, they will work with you.

- Bring back your stir-fry. There are many people who have gone from baby food to the grown up foods. There are many families that have stopped making basic recipes like chicken stir fry with broccoli or tomatoes with pasta and Parmesan. There are many exotic oils; as well as marinades so you are able to give these old basic recipes a great taste.

- Turn the electronic devices off when it is time for dinner. Enjoy your meals with family conversation and bonding time.

Chapter 4: Meal Planning and Recipes

It can be a little hard when you begin eating clean, in this chapter you will be given a meal plan along with the shopping list to make it even easier. The plan is for one week. This will make the transition a lot easier for you to handle.

Week One

- **Monday**:
  - ✓ **Breakfast**: Summer Omelet: Sauté 2 chopped green onions, ¼ cup of chopped fennel, 1 cup of chopped Swiss chard, 1 tbsp. of chopped dill, a dash of salt, and a dash of pepper with 2 tsp. of extra virgin olive oil. Add in four eggs; whisk them with 1 tsp. of water. Cook the egg and flip it once. Eat only half of the omelets and save the rest. Eat it with ½ cup of cherries and 1 slice of whole wheat bread.

  - ✓ **Snack**: 1 peach and ½ ounce of walnuts

  - ✓ **Lunch**: Halloumi Salad: Toss 2 ounces of grilled Halloumi that has been cubed ½ cup of chickpeas, ¼ cup of chopped cucumbers, and sliced tomatoes, 1 tbsp. of mint, dash of parsley and dash of dill. Add in 1 cup of arugula with 2 tsp. of extra virgin olive oil with some lemon juice. Add in a dash of salt and a dash of pepper. Serve it with three ounces of tuna.

- ✓ **Snack**: 2 tbsp. of Edamame hummus with ½ of cucumber cut into sticks.
- ✓ **Dinner**: 1 serving of curried apricot pan roasted chicken - eat half and save the rest

- **Tuesday**:
  - ✓ **Breakfast**: Strawberry Mint Smoothie: Blend 1 cup of kefir, 1 cup of strawberries, 2 Tbsp of mint, ½ cup of ice, 1 tsp. of honey, 1 tsp. of vanilla, 2 Tbsp of hemp seeds. Eat only half and freeze the rest into a Popsicle - Eat it with 1 slice of bread that has 2 Tbsp of peanut butter on it.
  - ✓ **Snack**: 2 Tbsp of Edamame hummus with ½ of a cucumber cut to sticks
  - ✓ **Lunch**: Summer Omelets - eat the leftovers with ½ cup of cooked farro and 1 peach
  - ✓ **Snack**: 1 ounce of walnuts and ½ cup of cherries
  - ✓ **Dinner**: Open Faced Veggie Melts and Smoked Mozzarella

- **Wednesday**:
  - ✓ **Breakfast**: Cherry Farro Parfait: In a parfait styled glass, layer in ⅔ cup of cooked farro, 1 Tbsp of chopped walnuts, ½ cup of sliced pitted cherries, ½ cup of kefir, 1 tsp. of hemp seeds, 2 tsp. of honey, and a dash of cinnamon, along with a dash of nutmeg.
  - ✓ **Snack**: 2 Tbsp of edamame hummus with ½ cup of fennel slices
  - ✓ **Lunch**: 1 serving of Curried Apricot Pan Roasted Chicken - leftovers

- ✓ **Snack**: 2 tsp. of peanut butter on top of ½ slice of bread. Sprinkle it with a dash of cinnamon and nutmeg after toasted.

- ✓ **Dinner**: Barramundi with Herb Sauce: Trim the asparagus bunch and then brush it with 2 tsp. of extra virgin olive oil, a dash of salt, and a dash of pepper. Grill it with zest from one lemon. Eat four of the spears and save the rest. Eat it with 1 cup of quinoa.

- **Thursday**:
  - ✓ **Breakfast**: Green Egg Benny: 4 asparagus spears that were leftovers, add in 3 slices of avocado topped with 1 egg over easy cooked in ½ tsp. of extra virgin olive oil. Drizzle it with ¼ of herb sauce leftovers.

  - ✓ **Snack**: Top ½ cup of kefir with ½ cup of sliced strawberries. Drizzle on 1 tsp. of honey.

  - ✓ **Lunch**: Strawberry Kale Salad: Toss in 2 cups of baby kale with ½ cup of sliced strawberries and cooked farro with 1 ounce of Halloumi, grilled and diced up. Add in 1 Tbsp of pistachios. Whisk 2 tsp. of extra virgin olive oil, 1 tsp. of balsamic vinegar, ½ tsp. of honey, dash of salt, and a dash of pepper. Drizzle on the salad. Eat it with 1 slice of whole wheat bread.

  - ✓ **Snack**: 2 tsp. of peanut butter on ½ of a sliced peach.

  - ✓ **Dinner**: 1 serving of curried apricot pan roasted chicken - leftovers

- **Friday**:
  - ✓ **Breakfast**: Avocado Mash with Hemp Seed: ¼ mashed avocado on top of 1 slice of bread, sprinkle it with 2 tsp. of hemp seeds, ¼ tsp. of lemon zest with a dash of salt and a dash of pepper. Eat it with a cup of cherries.
  - ✓ **Snack**:   tsp. of edamame hummus with four asparagus spears - leftovers
  - ✓ **Lunch**: Halloumi Salad: Toss 2 ounces of grilled Halloumi cubed with ½ cup of chickpeas, ¼ cup of cucumbers and sliced tomatoes, 1 Tbsp of chopped mint, dill, and parsley. Add in 1 cup of arugula with 21 tsp. of extra virgin olive oil and some lemon juice with a dash of salt and a dash of pepper. Serve it with 3 ounces of tuna. Eat the Popsicle.
  - ✓ **Snack**: ½ cup of sliced fennel drizzled with ¼ of herb sauce leftovers.
  - ✓ **Dinner**: Mediterranean Quinoa

- **Saturday**:
  - ✓ **Breakfast**: Strawberry Farro Bowl: 1 cup of cooked Farro with ½ cup of kefir, ½ cup of sliced strawberries, 2 Tbsp of chopped almonds, top it with 1 tsp. of honey and mint. Dash it with cinnamon and nutmeg.
  - ✓ **Snack**: ½ slice of bread with 2 tsp. of edamame hummus with ¼ cup of sliced cherry tomatoes
  - ✓ **Lunch**: Mediterranean Quinoa - leftovers
  - ✓ **Snack**: 1 ounce of walnuts with 1 orange
  - ✓ **Dinner**: grilled Steak and Romaine Hearts and Tangy Date Sauce

- **Sunday**:
  - ✓ **Breakfast**: Clean Green Scramble: Sauté 2 cups of kale in 2 tsp. of extra virgin olive oil, and 1 clove of minced garlic, 2 tsp. of chopped dill and parsley, 1 chopped green onion, a dash of salt, and a dash of pepper. Transfer it to a plate and then scramble 2 eggs inside the same pan. Eat it with ½ of a peach.

  - ✓ **Snack**: 1 cup of kefir with 1 ounce of toasted almonds. Sprinkle it with a dash of nutmeg and cinnamon. Eat it with ¼ cup of cherries

  - ✓ **Lunch**: Sea and Pea Salad: Combine 2 ounces of tuna with ½ cup of chickpeas, 1 chopped up green onion. ½ cup of chopped cucumber, and ½ cup of sliced tomatoes. Add in 2 tsp. of extra virgin olive oil, 1 tsp. of lemon juice, and 1 tbsp. of dill and parsley. Eat it with one slice of bread.

  - ✓ **Snack**: ½ slice of bread with 2 tsp. of edamame hummus and ¼ of the herb sauce.

  - ✓ Dinner: Mediterranean Quinoa - leftovers

Barramundi with Herb Sauce Recipe:

- Brush barramundi fillet with ½ tsp. of extra virgin olive oil.
- Sprinkle it with salt and some pepper.
- Grill is.
- In your blender, pulse in 1 clove of garlic, ¼ cup of extra virgin olive oil, 2 chopped green onions, juice from ½ lemon, and ⅓ cup of dill, parsley, and mint.
- Add in a dash of salt and a dash of pepper.
- Drizzle ¼ of the sauce on the fish and save the leftovers for the week.

Curried Apricot Pan Roasted Chicken and Broccoli Amandine

Ingredients:

- 4 - 5 ounce Chicken Breasts - Boneless and Skinless
- ⅛ tsp. of Sea Salt
- ⅛ tsp. of Pepper
- 3 Tbsp. of Olive Oil - Divided
- 2 Bunches of Broccoli - Trimmed
- 4 Green Onions - Chopped, Divided
- 2 Tbsp. of Ginger - Minced
- 2 Tbsp. of Garlic - Minced - divided
- 2 tsp. Of Curry Powder
- ½ tsp. of Red Pepper Flakes
- 4 Cups of Sliced Apricots - 8 Apricots
- ¼ cup of Dry White Wine
- ¾ Cup of Chicken Broth - Low Sodium
- 2 Tbsp. of Raw Honey
- Zest from ½ Orange
- 2 Tbsp of Unsalted, Organic Butter - Diced
- ¼ Cup of unsalted, Slivered Almonds

Instructions:

- Preheat your oven to 400 degrees Fahrenheit. Season your chicken with ⅛ tsp. of salt and pepper. In a large pan on high heat, heat up 2 tbsp. of oil. Add in the chicken and sear it until it is browned on both sides. It will take about four minutes. Flip it and transfer it to a pan for the oven. Roast it until it is cooked completely through. It will take about 10 minutes. Transfer it to a plate and add a foil tent.

- Blanch your broccoli in a pot of some boiling water until it is tender. It will take about 3-4 minutes. Drain it and transfer it to the ice water in order to cool. Drain it again and put it to the side.

- In the same pan with your chicken drippings on medium heat, add in whites of the green onions, the ginger, 1 tbsp. of garlic, curry powder and some pepper flakes. Seat it until the onions are soft. It will take about one minute.

- Stir in the apricots; increase your heat to med-high. Cover the pan and sauté it for 3 minutes. Add in the wince and scrape the browned bits from the pan using a wooden spoon. When the wine has evaporated, stir in the broth. Add in the honey and the orange zest. Cook it until the sauce thickens. It will take five to six minutes.

- Stir in the butter until emulsified. Stir in the greens of your onions; season it with a dash of salt and a dash of pepper. Cover it to keep it warm.

- In a large pan on medium heat, add in 1 tbsp. of oil. Add in 1 tbsp. of garlic and cook it for 30 seconds. Add in the broccoli and cook it until it is heated. It will take three minutes. Stir in the almonds and additional salt and pepper. Serve the sauce on the chicken and the broccoli on the side.

Mediterranean Quinoa and Red Beets

Ingredients:

- 1 cup of Quinoa - Rinsed
- 2 tbsp. of olive oil
- 3 cups of red beets - peeled, diced
- 1 bunch of green onions - sliced, divided white and green parts
- 2 tbsp. of garlic - minced
- 1 tbsp. of lemon zest - minced
- 2 tbsp. of lemon juice - divided
- 1 cup of parsley - chopped
- 1 cup of walnuts - toasted, chopped
- ¼ tsp. of sea salt
- ¼ tsp. of pepper
- Balsamic vinegar
- 6 tbsp. of feta cheese - crumbles

Instructions:

- In a large pan, cook the quinoa according to the instructions on the package. Transfer it to a bowl and put it aside.
- In the same pan on med-high heat your oil. Add in the beets and the whites of the onion. Sauté them until the beets are soft to a fork. It will take 10 minutes. Add in the garlic and cook it for 1 minute. Stir in the quinoa, onion greens, zest, and the juice. Add in the parsley and the walnuts. Season it with the salt, vinegar, and the pepper. Garnish it with 1 tbsp. of feta cheese.

Grocery List for Meal Plan

- *Proteins and Dairy*
  - ✓ 1 - 15 Ounce Barramundi Fillet
  - ✓ 4 - 5 Ounce Boneless, Skinless Chicken Breasts
  - ✓ 2 - 6 Ounces of Beef Tenderloin or Top Sirloin Medallions
  - ✓ 1 Dozen Eggs
  - ✓ 9 ounce BPA free canned or even Pouched Tuna - Ensure it is packed in water.
  - ✓ 1 quart of Plain Whole Milk Kefir
  - ✓ 5 Ounce Halloumi Cheese
  - ✓ 4 Ounces of Smoked Mozzarella Cheese
  - ✓ 2 Ounces of Feta Cheese
  - ✓ ½ Ounce of Shaved Parmesan Cheese
  - ✓ 8 Ounce Stick Organic Unsalted Butter

- *Whole Grains*:
  - ✓ 1 Bag of Quinoa
  - ✓ 1 Bag of Farro
  - ✓ 1 Package of Whole Rye Bread

- *Seeds, Nuts, and Oils*:
  - ✓ 1 bag of Hemp Seeds
  - ✓ ½ Ounce of Unsalted, Shelled Pistachios
  - ✓ 1 Jar of Unsalted Natural Peanut Butter
  - ✓ 3 Ounces of War Unsalted Almonds
  - ✓ 7 ½ Ounces of Raw Unsalted Walnuts
  - ✓ 1 Bottle of Extra Virgin Olive Oil
  - ✓ 1 Bottle of Olive Oil

- *Fruits and Vegetables*
    - ✓ 1 Large Avocado
    - ✓ 2 Cucumbers
    - ✓ 2 Fennel Bulbs
    - ✓ 3 Bunches of Green Onions
    - ✓ 1 Bunch of Asparagus
    - ✓ 1 Bunch of Fresh Mint
    - ✓ 1 Bunch of Fresh Dill
    - ✓ 1 Bunch of Fresh Parsley
    - ✓ 1 Large Head of Swiss Chard
    - ✓ 6 Ounces of Baby Kale
    - ✓ 2 Romaine Lettuce Hearts
    - ✓ 8 Ounces of Haricots Verts or Small Green Beans
    - ✓ 4 Lemons
    - ✓ 1 Pound of Beets
    - ✓ 1 Pint of Cherry Tomatoes
    - ✓ 3 Ounces of Arugula
    - ✓ 3 Bunches of Broccoli
    - ✓ 1 Yellow Bell Pepper
    - ✓ 2 - 1 Inch Pieces of Fresh Ginger
    - ✓ 1 Large Head of Fresh Garlic
    - ✓ 1 Pint of Strawberries
    - ✓ 13 ½ Ounces of Cherries
    - ✓ 2 Oranges
    - ✓ 8 Apricots
    - ✓ 4 Peaches
    - ✓ 12 Pitted Dates

- Extra:
  - ✓ 1 Bottle of Raw Honey
  - ✓ 1 Bottle of Pure Vanilla Extract
  - ✓ 1 Bottle of Balsamic Vinegar
  - ✓ 1 Bottle of Ground Cinnamon
  - ✓ 1 Bottle of Ground Nutmeg
  - ✓ 1 Bottle of Yellow Mustard Seeds
  - ✓ 1 Bottle of Sea Salt
  - ✓ 1 Bottle of Ground Black Pepper
  - ✓ 1 Bottle of Red Pepper Flakes
  - ✓ 1 Bottle of Dry White Wine
  - ✓ 1 Carton of Low Sodium of Chicken Broth
  - ✓ 1 Bottle of Curry Powder
  - ✓ 1 - 15 Ounces of BPA Free Chickpeas
  - ✓ 1 - 8 Ounce Container of All Natural Edamame Hummus

Chapter 5: Snacks for Clean Eating

Many people battle the typical hectic daily routines and when you want to eat clean, it can cause some more issues. However, in this chapter you are given clean eating snack ideas so you can prepare and be successful with your clean eating plans. Use this list as a guideline to stock your shelves and pantry to keep the clean eating going great.

- No-Bake Bars
- Peanut Butter Yogurt Dip and Fruit
- Carrots and Avocado Dip
- Asian Chicken and Vegetable Lettuce Wrap
- Peanut Butter Banana Cup
- Hard Boiled Eggs
- Cucumber and Tomato Salad
- Skinny Nutella
- Popcorn
- Apple Chips
- Berry Parfait
- Pineapple Spears
- Skinny Ranch Dip
- Fruit Popsicle
- Celery and Homemade Peanut Butter
- No-Bake Oatmeal Chocolate Chip Bites
- Sweet Potato Hummus and Whole Wheat Crackers

- Garden Salad
- Chili Lime Pumpkin Seeds
- Peanut Butter Honey Oat Bars
- Quinoa Crisps with Berry Parfait
- Sweet and Spicy Pecans
- Steel Cut Oatmeal
- Apple Nachos Supreme
- Simple Homemade Peanut Butter
- Roasted Red Pepper Hummus and Whole Grain Pita Chips
- Banana Blueberry Bars
- Cinnamon Honey Nuts
- Sweet Potato Fries
- Cranberry Pumpkin Seed
- Quinoa
- Skinny Ms. Granola
- Marinated Mushrooms
- Vegetable Soup
- Strawberry Banana Smoothie
- Baked Onion Rings
- Southwestern Kale Chips
- Belly Pepper Candy
- Sweet Potato Crunchies
- Watermelon and Red Onion Salad
- Skinny Ranch Dip with Broccoli
- Spinach Rolls and Ricotta and Pistachios
- Quinoa Protein Bars
- Oven Baked Sweet Potato Tots
- Lean Meatballs and Teriyaki Sauce
- Chocolate Peanut Butter Protein Smoothie

Chapter 6: Clean Eating Recipes

In this chapter you will be given recipes for clean eating during snack time, breakfast time, lunch, and dinner. We will begin with a generic shopping list. This is more of a master list that can be altered. As you move through the recipes, add the ingredients that you will need to the shopping list. Before you go to the grocery store, make sure that you eat a healthy snack. If you go to the store when you are hungry, you will have a harder time to stick to your clean eating diet.

Master Shopping List

Seafood and Meats
- Chicken Breasts
- Turkey Breasts
- Ground Turkey
- Ground Chicken
- Salmon, trout, halibut, mackerel, or other favorite seafood

Bread and Bakery
- Whole Wheat Bread
- Whole Wheat Pita Pockets
- Whole Grain Tortillas

Rice and Pasta
- Whole Wheat Pasta
- Brown Rice

Sauces, Oils, Dressings, and Condiments
- Tomato Sauce
- Barbecue Sauce
- Mustard
- Salsa
- Extra Virgin Olive Oil
- Canola Oil
- Jarred Olives
- Jarred Capers
- Hot Sauce

Breakfast Foods and Cereal
- Oatmeal
- Whole Grain Cereal Bars
- Whole Grain Cereal
- Multigrain Cereal

Canned Goods and Soup
- Diced Tomatoes
- Whole Peeled Tomatoes
- Salmon and Tuna Packed in Water
- Soups and Broth - Low Sodium
- Black Beans
- Kidney Beans
- Soy Beans
- Garbanzo Beans
- Lentils
- Split Peas
- Diced Green Chilies

Frozen Foods
- Broccoli
- Spinach
- Carrots
- Peas
- Strawberries
- Blueberries
- Raspberries
- Shrimp
- Low Fat Frozen Yogurt
- Whole Grain Waffles
- Whole Grain Vegetable Pizza

Cheese, Eggs, and Dairy
- Soymilk or Low Fat Milk
- Low Fat Yogurt
- Low Fat Cottage Cheese
- String Cheese
- Eggs
- Firm Tofu
- Organic Butter

Produce
- Bananas
- Oranges
- Apples
- Mangoes
- Blueberries
- Strawberries
- Sweet Potatoes
- Broccoli
- Baby Spinach
- Carrots

Crackers and Snacks
- Whole Grain Crackers
- Almonds
- Walnuts
- Cashews
- Pecans
- Peanuts
- Pistachios
- Dried Apricots
- Dried Figs
- Dried Prunes
- Raisins
- Dried Cranberries
- Sunflower Seeds
- Whole and Ground Flaxseeds
- Sesame Seeds
- Peanut Butter
- Soy Butter
- Almond Butter
- Hummus
- Dark Chocolate Pieces

Breakfast Recipes

Mixed Berry Cobbler:
- ½ cup of Almond, Coconut, or Hemp Milk
- ½ Cup of Blueberries
- ½ cup of Strawberries
- ½ cup of Blackberries
- 2 to 3 Medjool Dates
- Blend all of the ingredients together.

Tex Mex Style Scrambled Eggs:
- In a small pan, heat one tsp. of canola oil.
- Add in a corn tortilla and pan-fry it until it is crisp. It will take about two minutes.
- Remove it from the heat and dice it up.
- Sauté ⅛ of a jalapeno and ¼ cup of diced green and red bell peppers, tomato, and onion.
- Whisk 2 eggs and add them to the pan and scramble the eggs with the vegetables.
- Stir in the tortilla.
- Top it with 1 tbsp. of shredded cheese and 1 tbsp. of cilantro.

Egg in a Ring:
- Heat 1 tsp. of canola oil in a small pan on medium heat.
- Put one ¾ inch thick yellow or red bell pepper ring into the pan.
- Crack an egg into the middle of the ring and cook it until the white is firm.
- Flip it and cook it for another two minutes.
- Serve it with ¼ avocado, sliced thin and 1 slice of whole-wheat toast.

Vanilla Breakfast Pudding:

- Prepare 1 serving of cream of rice type cereal according to the instructions on the package. Keep out the salt.
- Whisk one egg in a small sized bowl.
- Whisk 2 tbsp. of cooked cereal into the egg, and then slowly whisk the egg mix into the cooked cereal.
- Add in ¼ tsp. of vanilla extract.
- Add in ¼ tsp. of cinnamon and 1 tsp. of sugar.
- Simmer it for 2 minutes.
- Top it with 2 tbsp. of chopped peaches.

Cheesy Easy Baked Egg

- Combine 1 tsp. of whole milk with ¼ tsp. of butter and 1 tsp. of grated Parmesan in a small sized bowl.
- Bring it to a boil.
- Crack 1 egg into the bowl and top it with 1 tbsp. of chopped tomato.
- Broil it until the white of the egg is set.
- Allow it to rest for 2 minutes.
- Sprinkle it with 1 tsp. of chives and 1 whole grain English muffin.

Clean Eating Lunch Recipes

These recipes can be used for dinner or snacks as well depending on what you like during certain times of the day. Another great idea is to double or triple the recipes so that you do not have to cook on a continuous basis. You will be able to stay with the clean eating plan.

Quinoa Fruit Salad and Honey Lime Vinaigrette
Ingredients:
- 1 Cup of Dry Quinoa - Pre-rinsed
- 2 Cups of Water
- ½ Cup of Blueberries - Fresh
- ½ Cup of Strawberries - Fresh
- ½ Cup of Mandarin Oranges
- ½ Cup of Mango Chunks
- 2 Tbsp. of Olive Oil
- Juice from 1 Lime
- 1 tsp. Of honey
- 1 Tbsp of Mint - Fresh, Chopped

Instructions:
- On med-high heat bring the water and the quinoa to a boil.
- Reduce the heat to low, cover it, and cook it for about 15 minutes or until your quinoa has absorbed most of the water.
- Turn off your heat and leave it covered for 5 minutes.
- Allow it to cool and then refrigerate it until it gets cold.
- Combine the quinoa with the fruit in a big bowl.
- Stir it to mix it.
- Add in the olive oil, honey, and the limejuice. Toss it with the salad and sprinkle on the mint.

Spring Greens and Strawberries with Candied Pecans

Ingredients:

- 4 cups of Spring Mix
- 2 Cups of Romaine Heart Lettuce - Tear to Bite Size
- 1 - 11 Ounce Can of Mandarin Oranges - Drained
- 1 Cup of Strawberries - Sliced
- 1 Small Sized Red Onion - Slice to Rings
- ½ Cup of Feta Cheese - Crumbled
- ½ Cup of Candied Pecans

Instructions:

- Combine all of the ingredients in a large sized salad bowl, drizzle on ½ cup of white balsamic vinaigrette or another salad dressing.
- Toss it to combine in.

Mediterranean Tuna Salad

Ingredients:

- 1 - 6 Ounce can of Tuna - Packed in Water
- ½ Cup of Artichoke Hearts - Diced
- ½ Cup of Kalamata Olives - Pitted, Chopped
- 1 Red Pepper - Roasted, Chopped
- ¼ Cup of Parsley - Chopped
- 2 tbsp. Of Basil
- 3 Tbsp of Olive Oil
- Juice from 1 Lemon
- Dash of Salt
- Dash of Pepper

Instructions:

- Combine all of you ingredients inside of a large sized bowl.
- Season it with salt and some pepper
- Chill it before you serve it.
- Serve the tuna salad on lettuce leaves, whole grain crackers, or a baguette.

Skinny Tacos in a Jar

Ingredients:

- ½ Pound of Turkey - Ground
- 1 tsp. Of Chili Powder
- ½ tsp. of Cumin
- ¼ tsp. of Garlic Powder
- ¼ tsp. of Sea Salt
- ½ Cup of Whole Grain Tortilla Chips - Broken
- ½ Cup of Shredded Cheese - Reduced Fat
- 3 Cups of Romaine Lettuce - Chopped
- 1 Cup of Cherry Tomatoes - Halved
- ½ Cup of Salsa - No Added Sugar

Creamy Salsa Dressing Ingredients:

- 2 Tbsp of Greek Yogurt
- 2 Tbsp of Mashed Avocado
- Juice from 1 Lime
- ¼ Cup of Salsa

Instructions:

- Heat a pan on medium heat and add in the turkey.
- Cook it until the turkey is no longer pink and it is cooked completely.
- Add the spices and stir it to combine it. Put it in a bowl and allow it to cool.
- In order to make the salad, divide the tortilla chips between six different jars.
- Layer each of them with half of the salsa, the turkey, tomatoes, the lettuce, and then the cheese.
- Make the dressing by blending the avocado, yogurt, limejuice, and the salsa in your blender.
- Blend it until it is smooth and creamy.
- Top the salad with some dressing, seal the jars and store the in your refrigerator until you are ready to eat it. It is good for two days.

Slow Cooker Minestrone

Ingredients:

- 1 Small Sized Onion - Diced
- 1 Celery Stalk - Diced
- 2 Carrots - Peeled, Sliced
- 1 Medium Sized Zucchini - Sliced
- 1 Large Sized Potato - Peeled, Cubed
- 2 Cups of Green Beans
- 1 Cup of Peas
- 2 Cups of Kale - Chopped
- 2 Cups of Vegetable Broth
- 1 - 15 Ounces of Diced Tomatoes - With Liquid
- 1 - 15 Ounce Can of Kidney Beans - Drained, Rinsed
- ½ Cup of Tomato Juice or Vegetable Juice
- 1 tsp. Of Sea Salt
- ¼ tsp. Of Pepper
- 4 Basil Leaves - Diced
- ½ Cup of Parmigiano Reggiano or Parmesan Cheese

Instructions:

- Add all of the ingredients to your slow cooker. Keep out the basil, kale, and the Parmesan.
- Cover it and cook it on low for 5-6 hours. You can cook it on high for 3-4 hours.
- When the minestrone is done, add in the kale. Put the lid back on it and allow the kale to wilt. It will take 5 minutes.
- Once it is ready to serve, drizzle a bit of extra virgin olive oil on the top of each bowl.
- Sprinkle it with the basil and the Parmesan.
- You are able to add one cup of whole-wheat penne pasta in the cooker for 30 minutes before the end of the cooking cycle.

Clean Eating Dinner Recipes

If you would like to prepare these recipes for another meal, they are great for lunches too. Just like the other meals, it is a good idea to double or triple the recipe in order to have leftovers to make things easier on you while you are transitioning to eating clean.

Quinoa Salad and Asparagus, Oranges, and Dates

Salad Ingredients:

- 1 tsp. of Olive Oil
- ½ Cup of White Onion - Chopped Fine
- 1 Cup of Quinoa - Uncooked
- 2 Cups of Water
- ½ tsp. Of Salt
- 1 Cup of Orange Sections
- ¼ Cup of Pecans - Toasted, Chopped
- 2 Tbsp. of Red Onion - Minced
- 5 Dates - Pitted, Chopped
- ½ Pound of Asparagus - Steamed, Chilled
- ½ Jalapeno Pepper - Diced

Dressing Ingredients:

- 2 Tbsp of Lemon Juice
- 1 Tbsp of Extra Virgin Olive Oil
- ¼ tsp. of Salt
- ¼ tsp. Of Pepper
- 1 Clove of Garlic - Minced
- 2 Tbsp of Mint - Chopped
- Mint Sprigs

Instructions:
- Prepare the salad: Heat 1 tsp. of oil in a large pan on med-high heat. Add in the white onion and sauté it for 2 minutes.
- Add in the quinoa to the pan. Sauté it for 5 minutes.
- Add 2 cups of water and ½ tsp. of salt into the pan. Bring it to a boil
- Cover it and reduce the heat to a simmer for 15 minutes.
- Remove it from the heat and allow it to stand for 15 minutes or until your water is absorbed.
- Transfer the quinoa mix to a large bowl. Add in the orange and the next 5 ingredients. Toss it gently.
- Prepare the dressing: Combine the juice and the following 4 ingredients in a small sized bowl.
- Stir it with a whisk.
- Pour the dressing on the salad. Toss it gently.
- Sprinkle the mint on top and garnish it with the mint sprigs.

Spinach and Fennel Salad with Shrimp and Balsamic Vinaigrette

Ingredients:
- 3 Slices of Bacon
- 1 Pound of Shrimp - Jumbo, Peeled, Deveined
- 2 Cups of Fennel Bulb - Sliced Thin
- 1 Cup of Grape Tomatoes - Halved
- ½ Cup of Sliced Red Onion
- 1 - 9 Ounce Package of Baby Spinach - Fresh
- 2 Tbsp. of Shallots - Chopped Fine
- 3 Tbsp. of Extra Virgin Olive Oil
- 1 Tbsp. of Balsamic Vinegar
- 1 tsp. Of Dijon Mustard
- ¼ tsp. Of Salt
- ¼ tsp. Of Pepper

Instructions:
- Cook the bacon in a pan on medium heat until it is crisp.
- Remove the bacon from the pan; keep the drippings and the crumbles.
- Add the shrimp into the pan. Cook it for 2 minutes. Turn it once.
- Combine the bacon, 2 cups of fennel, tomatoes, onion, and the baby spinach in a bowl.
- Combine the rest of the ingredients in a small sized bowl. Stir it with a whisk.
- Add the shrimp and the balsamic mix into the spinach mix. Toss it well.

Chicken and Brussels Sprouts with Mustard Sauce

Ingredients:

- 2 Tbsp. of Olive Oil - Divided
- 4 - 6 Ounces of Chicken Breast Halves - Skinless, Boneless
- ⅜ tsp. Of Salt - Divided
- ¼ tsp. Of Pepper
- ¾ Cup of Chicken Broth - Fat Free, Lower Sodium - Divided
- ¼ Cup of Apple Cider
- 2 Tbsp. of Dijon Mustard
- 2 Tbsp. of Butter - Divided
- 1 Tbsp. of Parsley - Chopped
- 12 Ounces of Brussels Sprouts - Trimmed, Halved

Instructions:

- Preheat your oven to 450 degrees Fahrenheit.
- Heat an ovenproof pan on high heat.
- Add in 1 tbsp. Of oil.
- Sprinkle the chicken with ¼ tsp. of salt and pepper. Add it to the pan.
- Cook it for 3 minutes or until it is brown.
  Turn the chicken. Place the pan inside the oven.
- Bake it for 9 minutes or until it is done.
- Remove the chicken fro the pan and keep it warm.
- Heat the pan on med-high heat.
- Add ½ cup of broth and cider. Bring it to a boil.
- Scrape the pan to loosen the brown bits.
- Reduce the heat to med-low heat. Simmer it for 4 minutes until it is thickened.
- Whisk in the mustard, 1 tbsp. butter, and the parsley.
- Heat the rest of the oil and 1 tbsp. of butter in a large pan on med-high heat.
- Add in the Brussels sprouts and sauté them for 2 minutes.
- Add in the rest of the salt and ¼ cup of broth into the pan. Cover it.
- Cook them for 4 minutes.
- Serve the sprouts with the chicken and the sauce.

Grape, Arugula, and Sunflower Seed Salad

Ingredients:

- 3 Tbsp of Red Wine Vinegar
- 1 tsp. of Honey
- 1 tsp. Of Maple Syrup
- ½ tsp. Of Mustard - Stone Ground
- 2 tsp. Of Grape seed Oil
- 7 Cups of Baby Arugula - Loosely Packed
- 2 Cups of Grapes - Red, Halved
- 2 Tbsp. of Sunflower Seed Kernels - Toasted
- 1 tsp. Thyme - Chopped
- ¼ tsp. Of Salt
- ¼ tsp. Of Pepper

Instructions:

- Combine the honey, vinegar, syrup, and the mustard in a small sized bowl. Gradually add in the oil. Stir it with a whisk.
- Combine the arugula, seeds, grapes, and the thyme in a large sized bowl.
- Drizzle the vinegar mix on the arugula.
- Sprinkle the salt and the pepper on the top.
- Toss it to coat it.

Lemon Chicken Kebabs and Tomato Parsley Salad

Ingredients:

- 3 Tbsp of Lemon Juice - Divided
- 1 Tbsp. of Garlic - Minced, Divided
- 1 ½ tsp. of Oregano - Dried, Divided
- ¾ tsp. of Pepper - Divided
- 3 Tbsp of Extra Virgin Olive Oil - Divided
- 4 - 6 ounces of Chicken - Skinless, Boneless, Cut to 1 ½ inch Cubes
- 2 Cups of Parsley Leaves - Fresh
- 1 Cup of Cherry Tomatoes - Chopped

Instructions:

- Combine the 2 tbsp. of juice, 2 tsp. of garlic, 1 tsp. of oregano, ½ tsp. of salt, and ½ tsp. of pepper in a bowl.
- Add in 1 tbsp. of oil; stir it with a whisk.
- Add in the chicken and stir. Marinate the chicken for 2 hours in the refrigerator covered.
- Remove the chicken from the bowl. Throw away the marinade.
- Thread the chicken on the skewers.
- Heat your grill pan on high heat.
- Add the skewers. Cook these for 6 minutes or until it is completely done. Turn it often.
- Combine the rest of the juice, garlic, oregano, salt, and the pepper in a medium sized bowl.
- Gradually add the rest of the oil and stir it well.
- Add in the parsley and the tomatoes. Toss it to coat it.
- Serve it with the chick on the top of the salad.

Conclusion:

Thank you again for purchasing this book!

I hope this book was able to help you to better understand what clean eating is and how you can get started without feeling overwhelmed.

The next step is to take note what you still have in your kitchen. As you run out of the items, replace them with organic and clean products. Instead of getting white rice, when you are out of white rice replace it with brown rice, and more.

Finally, if you enjoyed this book, please take the time to share your thoughts and post a review on Amazon. It'd be greatly appreciated!

Thank you and good luck!

Preview of The Sirtfood Diet

The Amazing Benefits of Activating Your Skinny Gene, including Recipes!

Chapter 1. What are Sirtfoods?

The Sirtfood Diet book was published in January, 2016. Authors of the book, Aidan Goggins and Glen Matten both have impressive credentials for writing and speaking about such an innovative area of health and nutrition.

Aiden is an Irish pharmacologist and Glen is from England. Both are experts in nutritional medicine. They jointly wrote another book a few years earlier as a critique on the supplement industry. Research on Sirtuins stemmed from their work, as a key to healthy weight and longevity.

Sirtuins are a family of proteins that are in living things, and are heavily involved in metabolic processes in the body. Sirtuins, to put it simply, will increase or decrease the way genes are expressed and then will impact what happens in the cell, tissues and organs. Sirtfoods are high in sirtuin, or more accurately, they are high in the activators of situins. They make them bloom and come alive.

Amidst the genetic molecular workings of situins, we are especially interested in how these compounds work to trigger fat-burning, to decrease weight, and to increase longevity. As you can see in the description, this is not just about a fad diet, but rather a researched base plan to get at the body's deeper processes related to our weight and our aging which are interrelated. An overweight body will age quickly. An aging body will not be able to optimize its metabolism and thus the cycle of aging continues.

There is a promise in consuming more Sirtfoods to activate the miraculous Sirtuins. The promise is in the evidence that Sirtfoods can help to increase or decrease these functions of the human body, and along with other healthy lifestyle habits, they will beneficially increase longevity and contribute to weight loss if these Sirtuins are activated.

Research also is being done of possible Sirtuin activator supplements, but supplements for Resveratrol (which will come up later in the book), which contribute to anti-aging as well, have shown to not be effective so the idea of supplements for Sirtuins is unknown. Many natural foods can easily activate Sirtuins, and this is the premise of the book. There are certain foods that are easily accessible to you, and in combinations, they will present the easiest and most natural ways to increase Sirtuin activation in your body, and to help your genes to express health and longevity.

The list of some known Sirtfoods that are the highest in Sirtuin compounds are below, in alphabetical order. Those foods with an asterisk have the highest levels, and are the most beneficial of all.

- Apples
- Aragula
- Blackcurrants*
- Capers*
- Celery
- Chicory (red)
- Chili pepper
- Citrus fruits
- Cocoa (fark chocolate)*
- Coffee
- Dates (Medjool)
- Extra virgin olive oil
- Fish oil (omega-3)*
- Green tea*
- Kale*
- Lavage
- Miso soup and other soy products
- Olives*
- Onions (red)*
- Parsley*
- Red wine
- Strawberries
- Tofu
- Turmeric*
- Walnuts

These foods are found in most grocery stores and in health food shops. They are not necessarily expensive either. A one-time fancy surf and turf dinner at a restaurant would cost much more than a bulk of money of these on a shopping list!